Fit Family Guide

A Parent's Roadmap to Wellness and Nutrition

Table of Contents

Chapter 1. Introduction

Welcome to our Special Report titled: "Fit Family Guide: A Parent's Roadmap to Wellness and Nutrition". Having a fit and healthy family isn't just about trips to the gym, it involves a diverse blend of smart nutrition and engaging physical activities that fit seamlessly into your daily routine. This report is a treasure trove of straightforward, science-driven advice that's designed to transform your family's health, relationships, eating habits, and overall lifestyle. Far from being a complicated tome, this guide is bursting with joy and vitality. It serves as your user-friendly passport to a world where wellness is fun, achievable, and becomes second nature! Make the choice to invest not just in this report, but in your family's future. Welcome to a whole new journey to wellness, wellness made fun, wellness made easy, and most importantly, wellness made for you and your loved ones.

Chapter 2. Understanding the Basics of Nutrition

Before diving into the abundant world of food and its influences on our physical health, understanding the basics of nutrition provides a strong foundation. By grasping these core principles, you can make informed decisions about what and when you and your family eat.

2.1. The Building Blocks of Food

All food consists of three primary macronutrients - carbohydrates, proteins, and fats - along with a range of micronutrients, such as vitamins and minerals. Understanding these components helps determine the potential benefits and pitfalls of different food choices.

Carbohydrates provide our bodies with their primary source of energy. Simple carbs, like sugars, offer quick spikes in energy but are short-lived, often leaving us feeling hungrier sooner. On the other hand, complex carbs, found in foods like whole grains, provide sustained energy as they are metabolically broken down slower.

Proteins are essentially the building blocks for virtually all of our body's tissues and organs. They play an essential role in building, maintaining, and repairing body tissue, and are also critical for enzyme and hormone function. Sources of protein include meat, fish, eggs, and plant-based alternatives like beans and lentils.

Fats have long been villainized in health discussions. However, healthy fats are an integral part of our diets. Fats provide a concentrated source of energy, support cellular growth, protect our organs, keep us warm, and aid in absorbing certain vitamins. Healthy fats are found in avocados, nuts, seeds, olives, and fish like salmon.

Micronutrients include vitamins and minerals, vital in keeping our bodies functional and well-oiled. Although needed only in small amounts, these mighty compounds maintain heart and bone health, secure our immunity, and participate in energy formation.

2.2. A Plate Model

A practical way to keep the principles of nutrition in mind while eating is to picture your plate. Half of the plate should be filled with fruits and vegetables for the fiber, vitamins, and minerals they offer. A quarter should be filled with whole grains - rich in fibers and complex carbs, while the remaining quarter is dedicated to proteins.

2.3. Meal Timing and Frequency

Despite popular belief, eating frequently does not necessarily boost metabolism. What matters most is the total caloric intake and expenditure in the day. For most families, having three balanced meals a day remains a practical strategy, with balanced snacks if required to maintain energy levels. Listen to your body's hunger and fullness cues, and try to make eating a mindful, intentional part of your day.

2.4. Understanding Food Labels

Food labels can unveil a product's true nutritional value beyond its marketing claims. The first item on the list is always the ingredient present in the largest quantity. Beware of hidden sugars, high sodium content, and unhealthy fats such as trans fats. Also, dietary fiber, vitamins, and minerals are nutrients you want to get more.

2.5. Nutritional Needs for Different Age Groups

Different family members will have different nutritional needs depending on their age, sex, activity level, and overall health status. Younger children have high needs for calcium and vitamin D for bone growth, teens need protein for growth spurts, and older adults may need more fiber to support digestive health.

2.6. Special Diets

There are numerous dietary patterns, from the Mediterranean diet to veganism, pescatarian, and gluten-free. All have their own benefits and considerations, and none is 'one-size-fits-all.' When making dietary changes, consider if they meet all nutritional needs and are feasible within your lifestyle.

2.7. Beware of 'Diet Culture'

Children are particularly sensitive to messages around food and body image. Avoid demonizing foods or promoting restrictive dietary practices. Instead, strive to promote a positive food environment, centered around nourishment, balance, and enjoyment, rather than guilt or rigid rules.

2.8. Hydration is Key

Although not a nutrient, water makes up around 60% of your body weight. It helps to flush out toxins, carry nutrients to your cells, and ensure optimal bodily function. Make a conscious effort to increase water intake, adding more if exercising or during hot weather.

By understanding the basics of nutrition, you equip yourself with the knowledge to guide your family towards a healthier, more balanced lifestyle. Remember that progress is more important than perfection, and there's always room for your family's favorite treats within a balanced diet. Gradually introducing these principles into your family life will turn them from conscious decisions into second nature, paving the way towards sustainable nutrition and overall wellness.

Chapter 3. The Wholesome Pantry: A Guide to Healthful Food Shopping

The path to a fit and healthy family starts right from your shopping cart. Every decision you make in grocery aisles contributes to the overall nutritional profile of your household. So, if you've ever wondered what essentials should be there in your pantry for a healthier lifestyle, you've come to the right place.

3.1. Understanding Nutrition Labels

As tedious as it might sound, understanding nutrition labels is the first step in healthful food shopping. There's more to it than simply checking the calorie count. Labels can contain a lot of information, but when you know how to read them, you can make the healthiest choices for your family.

1. Serving Size: The serving size is the first thing you'll see on a nutrition label. All of the information that follows is based on this portion size. Be careful not to assume that the whole package is a single serving!

2. Calories: The number of calories per serving is important to check, especially if you're trying to manage your family's weight.

3. Nutrients: Nutrients like fats, sodium, and sugars often come in larger amounts than needed in many packaged foods. Aim for low percentages of these nutrients.

4. Vitamins and minerals: High percentages of vitamins and minerals like Vitamin A, Vitamin C, calcium, and iron are a good sign.

Make label reading a family activity. Teaching children to understand these details can help foster healthy eating habits for a lifetime.

3.2. The Basics: Shop the Perimeter

The perimeter of most grocery stores is where fresh foods like vegetables, fruits, lean meats, fish, eggs, and dairy items are usually located. Starting your shopping excursion from the outer aisles ensures your cart fills up with whole, unprocessed foods first.

1. Fruits and Vegetables: Stock up on a variety of colorful fruits and vegetables. They are rich in fiber, vitamins, minerals, and antioxidants. Buying seasonal produce not only ensures optimal taste and nutrition but also cuts down on food miles.

2. Lean Proteins: Look for lean cuts of meat, poultry, and fish. Opt for skinless options whenever possible. Eggs, beans, and other plant-based proteins are also key to any balanced diet.

3. Dairy: When it comes to dairy and dairy alternatives, choose lower fat options where possible.

Remember, less processed is always better when it comes to healthy eating.

3.3. Essential Whole Grains

Whole grains should be a staple in any wholesome pantry. They contain many vitamins, minerals, and beneficial compounds that white, enriched grains do not. This includes fiber, B vitamins, and several minerals like zinc, iron, magnesium, and manganese.

1. Bread and Pasta: Opt for whole grain bread and pasta for their higher fiber content.

2. Rice: While white rice is not a bad choice, brown rice and wild rice have more fiber and more nutrients.

3. Oats: Rolled or steel-cut oats are a great breakfast staple. They are

rich in fiber, particularly soluble fiber, which helps keep your heart healthy.

Putting whole grains at the heart of your diet can contribute to improved digestive health, better heart health, and may help manage weight effectively.

3.4. Stock Up on Healthy Fats

Contrary to popular belief, not all fats are enemies of health. Monounsaturated and polyunsaturated fats, for example, can help reduce 'bad' LDL cholesterol levels and raise 'good' HDL cholesterol levels.

1. Nuts and Seeds: These small packets of nutrition contain a wealth of vital nutrients like protein, fiber, healthy fats, vitamins, and minerals.

2. Avocado: Avocado is rich in monounsaturated fats, fiber, and several vital vitamins and minerals.

3. Oils: Choose oils lower in saturated fats, such as olive, canola, or avocado oil.

It's important to incorporate some amount of healthy fats into your diet. They help in nutrient absorption, nerve transmission, and maintaining cell membrane integrity.

3.5. Limit Processed Foods and Sugars

While the convenience of processed foods is undeniable, they often come loaded with unhealthy additives, from high fructose corn syrup to trans fats. Save these foods for occasional treats and try not to make them staples in your pantry.

1. Sugary Drinks and Snacks: These often contain a large amount of added sugar, which can contribute to weight gain and other health problems.

2. Processed Meats: These products are usually high in sodium and saturated fats, and some contain nitrites and nitrates, which may pose health risks when consumed in high amounts.

3. Salty Snacks: While a little bit of salt is necessary in our diets, most of us consume far more than the recommended daily limit.

Healthy substitutions are available for almost all processed foods. And when you crave a sweet treat, fruits are an excellent alternative!

3.6. Meal Planning and Prep

Planning your meals in advance and preparing the ingredients will save you much time and hassle during the week. It will also help you stick to your nutritional goals.

1. Group Ingredients: Group ingredients that can be used in multiple meals throughout the week. You can roast or grill a large batch of vegetables, cook a pot of grains, or prep proteins like chicken or tofu ahead of time.

2. Organizing: Keep your pantry, fridge, and freezer organized. Label and date everything so you can keep track of your inventory.

3. Cook in Batches: If you have time, cook meals in large quantities and freeze in portions.

Remember, the key to successful meal prepping is being creative and making sure your meals stay tasty and exciting.

A well-stocked pantry can be the backbone of a healthy diet and can make meal preparation a much more enjoyable experience. Every choice you make while shopping can ultimately reflect on your family's health and wellbeing. So, invest time in understanding what goes into your food and make choices that value nutrition and taste.

Chapter 4. Cooking up Fitness: Tasty and Nutritious Recipes

Let's dive in with open minds and empty stomachs, eager to explore the delectable journey of fit and healthy cooking. The kitchen is a wonderful place to foster wellness, it's where wholesome food, creativity, and family bonding intersect.

4.1. Understanding Nutritional Needs

Firstly, understanding nutritional needs is paramount. Embarking on this journey shouldn't mean foregoing all your family's favourite foods. By grasping the basic principles of nutrition, we can tweak beloved recipes for healthier versions without sacrificing taste.

The five primary nutrients our bodies need are carbohydrates, proteins, fats, vitamins, and minerals.

Carbohydrates: They are the body's primary source of energy. Opt for complex carbs like whole grains, veggies, and fruits which keep you feeling fuller for longer.

Proteins: Vital for growth and repair of body tissues. Lean meats, fish, eggs, dairy, and plant-sources like beans or soy can supply your protein needs.

Fats: These are concentrated sources of energy, with unsaturated fats being the healthiest choice. Foods like olive oil, avocados, and nuts are excellent sources.

Vitamins & Minerals: Found in fruits, vegetables, dairy products, and meats, these are needed in small quantities but are crucial for various body functions.

Fibre: Last but not least, don't forget about dietary fibre, an important nutrient that aids digestion and keeps you feeling satiated.

4.2. The Art of Meal Planning

Meal planning is the cornerstone of fit nutrition. It saves time, money, reduces food waste, and disallows unhealthy, impulsive meal choices. Start by planning your weekly meals, including breakfast, lunch, dinner, and snacks. Consider your family's food preferences, dietary restrictions, and the ingredients you have on hand. Remember, simplicity is key. Aim for meals that are quick, convenient, and bursting with nutritional goodness.

4.3. Kid-friendly Recipe Ideas

Creating meals that are not just nutritious but also kid-friendly can be a tough task. Here are a few ideas which can help you pull off this feat:

1. Whole Grain Pancakes: Substitute regular flour with whole grain flour. These pancakes are a perfect breakfast meal - couple them with honey, yogurt, or fresh fruits for added taste and health.

2. Veggie-loaded Pizza: Make your pizza dough using whole wheat and top it with a rainbow of veggies and lean meats. Pair with homemade tomato sauce and a sprinkle of cheese for a movie night favorite.

3. Healthy Tacos: Opt for lean proteins like chicken, fish, or beans as your fillings. Incorporate lettuce, tomatoes, and avocados for a fresh crunch. Corn tortillas or whole grain shells are a healthier choice compared to the regular flour ones.

4.4. Slash the Sugar

Reducing sugar intake is a key aspect of a healthy lifestyle. You can substitute white sugar with healthier alternatives like honey, agave nectar, or stevia in your recipes. Experiment with spices like cinnamon or nutmeg to ramp up the flavor while reducing sugar. Remember, limiting packaged foods can significantly cut down added sugars in your family's diet.

To help you out, here's a recipe that is delicious with natural sweetness.

1. Sweet Potato Muffins: Use boiled and mashed sweet potatoes, whole grain flour, honey, and a dash of cinnamon to bake a delicious batch of muffins. This mildly sweet treat is perfect for an afternoon snack or dessert.

4.5. Hydrate the Healthy Way

Finally, let's not forget about beverages. Most fruit juices and soft drinks are loaded with sugars and offer almost no essential nutrients. Instead, encourage your family to hydrate with water, milk, 100% fruit juices, and homemade smoothies. To make your water more fun, add slices of lemons, cucumbers, or various berries.

Now that we've toured through the vast landscape of nutrition, let's remember that balance is the key and the journey to fitness is one meal at a time. Next time you find yourself in the kitchen, see it as more than just a place to cook meals. See it as your family's health lab, where each ingredient and recipe becomes an essential formula in the science of your family's wellbeing.

Chapter 5. Decoding the Science of Exercise for All Ages

Understanding the importance of regular physical activity for all ages is crucial in the pursuit of holistic family wellness. Bounding with energy when we're young, transitioning into different exercise expectations during adulthood, and navigating the complications of maintaining physical activity later in life, the journey of exercise is one that transforms as continuously as we do.

5.1. The Significance of Exercise

Exercise crucially bolsters our health in a number of different ways, irrespective of age. It strengthens the heart and lungs, increases energy levels, helps to maintain a healthy weight, fosters better sleep, sharpens the mind, supports healthy muscles and bones, and contributes positively to overall emotional wellbeing. By breaking this down further and understanding the nuances within each age group, we can more effectively promote physical fitness throughout the lifespan.

5.2. The Early Years: Exercise for Children

For children, physical activity is not just about promoting growth and development but also about instilling a sense of joy in being active. Children as young as 3 years old can participate in regular physical activity. Focus should be more on play-based activities that enhance gross motor skills, balance, coordination, and agility.

Activities may include playing tag, playing on jungle gyms, simple gymnastics, swimming, or riding a bike. Schools and society should aim to encourage one hour of exercise each day for young children.

Table. Recommended Physical Activities for Children

Age	Activity
3-5	Playground play, swimming, dancing, cycling
6-9	Team sports e.g., basketball, soccer, swimming, cycling, martial arts
10-13	Endurance and strength activities (mosquito disruptions), team sports, martial arts, swimming, outdoor adventure activities

Remember, the focus is on creating a fun atmosphere where the child is excited about physical activity, not just treating it like a chore.

5.3. Adolescence: Transition and Transformation

With age, physical activity becomes more structured and can be an outlet for the torrent of changes that occur during adolescence, both physically and emotionally. Regular exercise during these years can help tackle issues like obesity, improve self-esteem, reduce stress and anxiety, and boost academic performance.

Your teenager might already have interests in specific sports or activities. Encourage these, but also make them aware of the importance of general fitness. Activities should now aim at improving cardiovascular fitness, strength, flexibility, and body composition. Hence, there can be a gradual move from spontaneous play to more organized and structured forms of exercise. It could also be beneficial for adolescents to engage in resistance training with appropriate guidance and supervision.

Table. Recommended Physical Activities for Adolescents

Age	Activity
14-19	Aerobic exercise (running, swimming), strength training (with supervision and guidance), team sports, outdoor adventure activities

5.4. Adulthood: Balancing Health and Lifestyle

In adulthood, where responsibilities often take precedence, and lifestyle diseases start to peek around the corner, regular exercise becomes even more crucial. Aim for at least 150-300 minutes of moderate intensity aerobic activities or 75-150 minutes of vigorous intensity activities per week, coupled with strength training activities on two or more days a week.

Table. Recommended Physical Activities for Adults

Age	Activity
20-64	Aerobic exercise (running, swimming, cycling), strength training, team sports, outdoor adventure activities, yoga, pilates

While it can be hard to fit in, creative solutions like walking or biking to work, exercise breaks during the workday, or family activities can help squeeze in the required exercise.

5.5. The Golden Years: Exercise for Seniors

Exercise in the golden years can help manage chronic health problems, improve balance, coordination, motor control, and maintain cognitive function. Being physically active can also enhance mood, well-being, and overall quality of life in older adults.

Senior-friendly activities like walking, swimming, gentle yoga, or tai chi are excellent. Additionally, strength training, flexibility, and balance exercises are also beneficial.

Table. Recommended Physical Activities for Older Adults

Age	Activity
65+	Walking, swimming, gentle yoga, tai chi, resistance training, balance exercises

Despite the compelling data showing the benefits of physical activity in all age groups, getting started and maintaining a regular exercise routine can be daunting. Hence, creating a supportive, family-centric environment for exercise, where everyone can participate and enjoy physical activity, is the key to long-term adherence. Ensuring games for children that is fun, adventure activities for teenagers that are thrilling, engaging activities for adults that can be merged into everyday life, and activities for seniors that can help them maintain a fit and healthy lifestyle can not just create a healthier family but a happier one.

In essence, fitness is not one size fits all. Just like we adapt and evolve, so should our approach to exercise. By decoding the science of exercise across all ages, we equip ourselves with the knowledge and understanding to make healthier, more informed choices for ourselves and our loved ones.

Chapter 6. Family Friendly Physical Activities: Making Fitness Fun

Incorporating regular and enjoyable physical activities into your family's routine is one of the most effective strategies to foster fitness and wellness. But how can you turn exercise into an appealing pastime, rather than a obligatory chore? Let's dive into effective methods to make physical fitness fun and fulfilling for your family.

6.1. Design Dynamic and Enjoyable Workouts

Activity and exercise shouldn't be mundane; rather, they ought to be unpredictable, engaging, and customizable. And yes, they should definitely be fun! Our bodies need an assortment of exercises to help engage different muscle groups, boost cardiovascular health, increase flexibility, and enhance overall strength. Here are a few ways to turn up the fun factor on family fitness:

- Merge Entertainment and Exercise: Why not make a game out of fitness? Invent engaging activities that stimulate both the mind and body. This could be as simple as a dance-off to your favorite tracks or a family-wide hula-hoop competition. The key is to cultivate an atmosphere of laughter and camaraderie, to help your family connect exercise with enjoyment.

- Organize Themed Workout Days: Devote specific days to unique styles of movement. Maybe Mondays are for yoga, while Fridays are for family soccer matches. Creating diversity in your routine helps prevent workout boredom and keeps everyone excited about what's next.

- Incorporate Technology: With a wealth of fitness apps and online games available, technology can be a powerful accomplice in your fight for fitness. Use fitness apps designed to gamify exercise or online workout tutorials to keep your family moving.

6.2. Outdoor Activities: The Perfect Blend of Fitness and Fresh Air

One of the prime ways to infuse fitness with fun is by taking advantage of the boundless opportunities provided by the great outdoors. Nature's playground offers a variety of ways to keep your family fit while basking in fresh air and sunlight, shown to improve mental health as well as physical well-being.

- Plan Regular Excursions: Make the most out of weekends or school holidays by scheduling regular outdoor adventures. This could be anything from mountain hikes, beach days, bicycling trips, or camping journeys. Each adventure offers plenty of opportunities for physical activity, while the change of scenery offers mental refreshments.

- Instigate Neighborhood Games: Encourage your family to participate in neighborhood sports matches, or organize your own. These can take the form of softball tournaments, cricket games, or touch football matches. Not only do such activities promote physical fitness, but they also help to foster community spirits and friendships.

- Gardening Wonders: Engage your children in the process of planting and maintaining a garden. This activity is excellent for teaching them about nature, nutrition, and the value of hard work while also serving as a light form of exercise!

6.3. Get Creative with Indoor Activities

Not every day will boast an idyllic outdoor weather, but a gloomy day doesn't have to mean a sedentary day. Here are some creative ways to keep the blood pumping indoors:

- Indoor Obstacle Course: Transform your living room into an obstacle course that will bring the whole family off the couch and onto their feet. Use pillows, furniture, and household items to create different challenges. Make sure the course is safe and age-appropriate for all players.

- Fitness Challenges: Hold an impromptu push-up, sit-ups, or jumping jacks contest. You can craft a leaderboard and track progress over the weeks. The element of competition can become a potent incentive to keep moving.

- Virtually there: Explore the fantastic world of fitness oriented video games. Whether it's dancing, training for martial arts, or virtually jogging through a scene straight out of a sci-fi movie, these games can make exercise exhilarating and engaging.

6.4. Incorporate Activity into Routine Tasks

Some of the best opportunities to enhance fitness levels come by making everyday tasks more physically active:

- Active Transport: Encourage walking or cycling to school or work, if feasible and safe. Biking or walking, even partway, can contribute significantly towards your daily recommended physical activity.

- Do Chores Together: Create a habit of doing household chores together. Chores like sweeping, vacuuming, gardening, or washing the car can also serve as subtle physical activities.

- Stretch During Screen Time: If your family is watching a show or a movie, use the commercials or intermission for a quick stretch or mini workout. This can help to break up long periods of inactivity and keep your family alert.

Taking steps to infuse fun into family fitness not only benefits the physical health of each family member, it can also enhance emotional bonds, improve mental health, and create lifelong memories. The key is to keep the activities diverse and appealing, regularly alternating and upgrading your fitness routine. physical fitness consistent, diverse, and fun. And remember, every step counts, every movement matters, and every laugh makes it all the more worthwhile.

Because in the end, wellness isn't just a journey, it's a lifestyle. And what better way to embrace it than with the shared joy and encouragement of family fitness.+=

Chapter 7. A Beginner's Guide to Mindful Eating

The path to better health and wellness often begins with mindful eating, the practice of paying attention to the sights, smells, textures, and tastes of your food, as well as your hunger and fullness cues. It's about appreciating meals as not just fuel for the body, but also an opportunity for well-being, satisfaction, and joy.

7.1. Understanding Mindful Eating

Mindful eating is not a diet, but a practice. It involves focusing your full attention on your food, appreciating its complexities and tuning into your internal signals of hunger and satiety. Rather than rapid, distracted eating, a mindful eater savors each mouthful of food, engaging all their senses to fully experience the act of eating.

7.2. The Power of Mindful Eating

Mindful eating has immense potential to transform your relationship with food and subsequently, your health. It aids weight regulation, promotes an improved relationship with food, lowers stress levels, fosters greater enjoyment of meals, and may even reduce symptoms of certain chronic conditions.

7.3. The How of Mindful Eating

1. Tune into hunger: Pay attention to your body's signals. Instead of eating on a schedule, eat when you're truly hungry.

2. Make mealtime special: Set the table, light a candle - make your meal an event. This underscores the importance of feeding your body with nourishing food.

3. Chew thoroughly: This aids digestion, and gives you enough time to appreciate flavors and textures.

4. Savor your food: Don't rush; take time to eat slowly. Your body takes about 20 minutes to register fullness.

7.4. Benefits of Mindful Eating

Mindful eating supports a healthy relationship with food by focusing on the quality rather than the quantity of food. Here are some benefits:

1. Weight Control: It encourages slower, more thoughtful eating - allowing time for satiety signals to kick in.

2. Improved Digestion: Chewing food thoroughly and eating slowly helps digestion.

3. Stress Reduction: Focusing solely on your meal helps to lower stress by drawing your attention away from worries.

4. Better Control over Eating Habits: It promotes listening to your own body's cues about hunger and fullness rather than following external rules about what and when to eat.

7.5. Mindful Eating and Children

Teaching kids mindful eating is a wonderful gift that could lead to healthier eating patterns as they grow into adults.

1. Set the example: When adults practice mindful eating, they set an example for children to follow.

2. Make meals a family affair: Make mealtime a shared, enjoyable experience. This can foster a lifelong appreciation for mindful eating.

3. Encourage exploration: Provide a variety of healthy foods for children to explore, savor, and enjoy.

7.6. The Challenges of Mindful Eating

Adopting mindful eating can be challenging in a fast-paced, convenience-oriented world that often prioritizes speed and efficiency over time spent preparing and savoring meals.

1. Patience: Mindful eating requires practice and patience as you learn to slow down and tune into your body's cues.

2. Finding Time: Preparing and enjoying a meal mindfully can be a challenge when time is tight.

3. Overcoming Habits: Habits such as eating in front of a screen can be hard to break.

7.7. Overcoming the Challenges

1. Start small: Begin by practicing mindful eating during one meal per day.

2. Get the family involved: Encourage every family member to participate. This makes it more enjoyable and can fortify the practice of mindful eating within your routine.

3. Seek support: If you're finding it tough, attending mindfulness classes or seeking help from a registered dietitian can be beneficial.

Remember, change takes time and patience. Celebrate each small achievement and be kind to yourself. Mindful eating isn't about perfection. It's a journey of self-discovery, appreciation, and ultimately, better health.

Chapter 8. You Are What You Drink: The Importance of Hydration

In understanding the significance of hydration, we must first appreciate the role fluids play in our bodies. From filling cells to aiding digestion, from flushing waste to temperature regulation, water's influence on our health is all-encompassing. Shortages of this vital fluid, on the other hand, can lead to dehydration, a condition that can range from mild discomfort to, in extreme scenarios, a life-threatening emergency. Here, we spotlight the importance of hydration, particularly the healthy choices you can make to maintain it.

8.1. The Role of Water in Our Bodies

Water makes up approximately 60% of an average adult's body weight, and an even higher percentage in children. It's essential in various physiological processes, including digestion, absorption, transportation of nutrients, and elimination of body wastes.

Every system in our body needs water. For example, our brain relies on a balanced water supply to function correctly. Even a minor degree of dehydration can lead to headaches, lack of concentration, and reduced cognitive function. In comparison, our cardiovascular system requires sufficient hydration for blood circulation, carrying oxygen, and essential nutrients to every cell.

8.2. The Consequences of Poor Hydration

Inadequate intake of water can quickly lead to dehydration, depicted by symptoms such as dizziness, fatigue, and confusion. Chronic dehydration can have more serious health effects, making it crucial to ensure an adequate intake of water daily.

Dehydration can impact physical performance significantly. Even a 2% decrease in body water can lead to a noticeable decline in physical performance, more so in hot environments.

8.3. The Hydration Equation: How Much Water Do You Need?

Not everyone's hydration needs are the same. They can differ based on factors such as age, climate, physical activity, and overall health.

A general rule is striving for eight 8-ounce glasses of water each day (the 8×8 rule), but this guideline may fall short for those living in hot climates or participating in strenuous exercise. An adult male living in a temperate climate and getting the recommended amount of moderate exercise might need closer to 13 cups of water per day, while an adult female might require about 9 cups.

8.4. Healthy Fluid Intake: It's More Than Just Water

While water is vital, other fluids can contribute to your hydration. These include beverages like milk, herbal teas, and fruit juices. Furthermore, approximately 20% of your daily hydration requirement can be satisfied by water-rich foods like cucumbers, tomatoes, watermelons, and oranges. However, one needs to be mindful of the sugar content in certain fruit juices and drinks.

8.5. Hydration for Kids

Keeping children hydrated can sometimes prove challenging. The introduction of flavored water, or infusing water with their fruit of choice, makes water consumption more appealing. Cultivate the habit of carrying a water bottle during outdoor activities.

The hydration needs of children vary based on their age, weight, and sex. For instance, a toddler might require 1.3 liters of fluid compared to the 1.7 liters that slightly older children need.

8.6. Caffeine and Alcohol: Hydrating or Dehydrating?

Though it's a popular belief that coffee and other caffeinated drinks are dehydrating, moderate amounts do not significantly affect hydration. However, at higher levels, caffeine can have a diuretic effect.

Alcohol, on the other hand, acts as a diuretic and can lead to increased fluid loss. It's best to limit consumption and remember to drink water in-between alcoholic beverages to mitigate the dehydrating effects.

8.7. Hydration for Physical Activity

Staying hydrated becomes particularly vital during exercise. As our bodies perform strenuous activity, we lose more water via sweat, and not replenishing this lost water can lead to fatigue and decreased performance.

Check your body weight before and after exercise. For each pound lost during activity, aim to consume around 16 to 24 ounces of water. Consuming sports drinks with electrolytes can be beneficial during long periods of high-intensity exercise.

By understanding the significant role water plays in our health and the serious impacts of poor hydration, families can make more informed choices about their fluid intake. Making hydration a priority is a simple, daily practice with long-lasting benefits. Ranging from enhanced mental clarity and mood to better physical performance and digestion, getting enough water is an essential component of overall wellness.

Chapter 9. De-Stress and Unwind: Family Wellness beyond Food and Fitness

The frenetic rush and hustle of our daily lives can cause an unhealthy level of stress that seeps into our homes. While proper nutrition and regular exercise are essential components of wellness, they are only part of the equation. This chapter delves into the equally vital areas of mental and emotional well-being, building strong and healthy relationships, and fostering a tranquil and supportive home environment.

9.1. Creating a Calm Home Environment

Harmony within the home is a foundational pillar of wellness. An environment filled with anxiety and tension detracts from our well-being and ability to manage stress effectively. Making your home into a haven of tranquility can go a long way in promoting the overall wellness of each family member.

One of the simplest, yet effective ways to foster a calm home environment is through organization. Clutter not only muddles our physical space but also our mental state. A clean, well-organized home reduces stress, facilitates efficiency, and enhances our mood.

Set aside time each week for a family cleaning event and execute it as a team action rather than an individual task. Make it fun, with playlists and friendly competitions. Not only will this result in a tidier space, but it also promotes cohesion and teamwork.

9.2. The Art of Mindfulness

Mindfulness, the practice of focusing on the present moment, is known to reduce stress and improve mental well-being. Encouraging each family member to develop mindfulness can have wide-ranging benefits, from increased concentration and improved sleep to a greater sense of peace and contentment.

Daily family mindfulness activities could include meditation, mindful walks, or practicing yoga together. Conversations during meals could solely center around the sensory experience, training everyone to stay present and avoid distracted eating.

Importantly, normalising quiet time where each person can reflect on their thoughts and feelings fosters an atmosphere where thoughts and emotions are not something to be feared or avoided, but acknowledged and understood.

9.3. Nurturing Positive Interactions

The family dynamic significantly impacts mental and emotional health. Prioritize positive, loving, and respectful communication. Research shows that families who share meals regularly enjoy better relationship quality and improved physical and mental health. Make meal times an electronic-free zone, encourage sharing of thoughts, celebrate successes, and openly discuss challenges.

Family bonding activities such as board game nights, weekly hikes, or crafting sessions contribute towards building strong relationships and developing shared memories. Acts of kindness and recognition of each other's accomplishments creates a culture of positivity.

9.4. The Importance of Downtime

Downtime is essential for rejuvenating the mind and body. Whether it's reading a book, pursuing a hobby or simply taking a nap, having regular downtime can greatly reduce stress levels and improve overall mood.

Aim to have a family "quiet hour" each day where everyone engages in their choice of low-key, relaxing activity. Such timeouts allow the brain to reset, promoting creativity, problem-solving abilities, and emotional well-being.

9.5. Cultivating Emotional Resilience

Building emotional resilience in the family enables each member to effectively handle stress and recover from adversity. Regular discussions about feelings, empathy, and managing emotions are important.

Look for teachable moments in everyday life where you can talk about feelings and emotions. Encourage your children to express their emotions promoting emotional intelligence from a young age. Highlight the importance of empathy by demonstrating it in your interactions.

9.6. Promoting Healthy Sleep Habits

Quality sleep is vital to stress management and overall health. Ensure your home promotes healthy sleep habits. Establish consistent sleep-wake schedules, limit evening screen time, and create calming pre-bedtime routines.

Taking a holistic approach to wellness, including mental and emotional aspects can effectively reduce stress levels and promote overall family well-being. By creating a calm and nurturing home environment, cultivating mindfulness, promoting positive interactions, prioritizing downtime, fostering emotional resilience, and maintaining healthy sleep habits, you can ensure a roadmap toward a healthy and happy family.

Chapter 10. Creating Sustainable Wellness Habits

Investing effort into the creation of sustainable wellness habits can undoubtedly have lifelong positive impacts on the health and wellbeing of your family. Forming these habits takes time, consistency, and a lot of patience, but the effort is more than worth it, especially when considering the improved physical, mental, and emotional health it brings to each member of your family.

10.1. Habit Formation and Sustainability

Habits shape us to a massive extent. They account for about 40 percent of our behaviors on any given day. In a wellness journey, habit formation is an uphill battle worth fighting, but the key to this fight lies in understanding the habit loop. This loop consists of the cue, the routine, and the reward. The cue triggers the brain to initiate the behavior, the routine is the behavior itself, and the reward is what the brain receives after the behavior, which helps it remember the habit loop in the future. The loop — Cue, Routine, Reward — is a key component in creating sustainable habits.

To build a new habit, you need to introduce a new cue, establish a routine around it, and reinforce it with a positive reward. Like building a muscle, forming new habits will take consistent work, but the more frequently you perform this action, the easier it will get. Consistency drives habit formation, and understanding this will be a vital tool in our journey towards a healthier family lifestyle.

10.2. Making Wellness a Family Affair

Getting all members involved in wellness activities enhances the success of forming sustainable habits. You could begin by establishing a 'Family Wellness Hour', during which everyone engages in a physical activity, or cooks a healthy meal together. This shared experience not only strengthens your shared commitment to wellness but also improves your familial bonds.

Consider creating a 'Family Wellness Plan' where all family members have input in setting wellness goals, meal planning, and fitness activities. This aids in creating a sense of responsibility and accountability for their health and encourages active participation in maintaining it.

10.3. Incorporating Physical Activities

Remember that physical activities should be fun and varied to hold your family's interest. Walking, cycling, swimming, dancing, sports are all excellent activities for incorporating movement into your daily routine. Consider integrating fitness prompts into your schedule — taking the stairs instead of the elevator, parking further away to walk a distance, or even a quick yoga session during a TV commercial break!

Regular physical activity is also necessary to stave off chronic diseases and maintain a healthy weight. A good guideline is at least 150 minutes of moderate aerobic activity or 75 minutes of vigorous activity every week, along with strength training exercises twice a week.

10.4. Building a Culture of Healthy Eating

Nutrition builds the foundation of wellness. Start with small steps such as reducing the intake of processed foods and incorporating more fresh fruits and vegetables into your diet. Acknowledge your kids' small victories when they opt for healthy choices, such as choosing a piece of fruit over a sugary snack.

Mealtime is also an opportunity for socializing and reconnecting. Make it a rule to have at least one meal together as a family each day. This won't just promote healthy eating habits but will also strengthen your family bonds.

10.5. Making Sleep a Priority

A healthy lifestyle isn't complete without enough restorative sleep. Establish a consistent bedtime routine that promotes quality sleep, and lead by example. Children and adults have different recommended amounts of sleep, but what's important is to ensure that each family member is getting the amount they need.

10.6. Mindfulness, Stress Management, and Mental Wellness

Encouraging mindfulness goes a long way in sustainable wellness. Simple activities such as breathing exercises, meditation, or time spent in nature can help reduce anxiety and unwanted stress.

Remember that emotional and mental wellness is as important as physical wellness. Create an open environment where family members can talk freely about their feelings and stresses. This includes developing good listening habits, empathetic behavior, and mutual respect within the family.

10.7. Consistent Health Checks

Scheduling regular health check-ups can help preempt potential issues and manage existing ones. Inculcate this practice early in life, which will allow children to grow up seeing it as part of their overall wellness plan.

10.8. Celebrate Progress, Not Perfection

Most importantly, remember to celebrate progress, however small it may be. The journey to sustainable wellness is not about unrealistic perfection; it's about making incremental improvements that over time accumulate to create massive health benefits.

Creating sustainable wellness habits means integrating wellness into your family's everyday life while making it enjoyable and achievable. By following these guidelines, your family will grow stronger, healthier, and happier, reaping the benefits of a fit lifestyle now and well into the future. Remember, wellness isn't a destination, but a journey that your family embarks on together, supporting and strengthening each other along the way!

Chapter 11. Charting Your Family's Health Progress: From Measurement to Motivation

Creating and sustaining a thriving, healthy family environment requires systematic planning, tracking, and motivation. Having an efficient and functional roadmap to monitor your family's health can significantly transform your wellness journey. This comprehensive guide walks you through the various aspects of assessing your family's health progress, encouraging motivation, and maintaining consistency.

11.1. The Importance of Measurement

A transformation journey begins by knowing your 'starting point.' Before embarking on your fitness quest, it's vital to measure each family member's health status. Health metrics spanning from body mass index (BMI), blood pressure, heart rate, cholesterol levels, to stamina constitute an overall health picture. Not only do these measurements serve as baseline figures for future comparison, but they allow for specific, personalized goals for every family member.

It is also noteworthy because of how these metrics interplay with clinical health risks. For instance, high cholesterol levels or high blood pressure may signal heart disease risks. Awareness and timely interventions can thus prevent or manage potential health crises.

11.2. Establishing Health Metrics

Setting up practical health metrics requires you to consider a few factors. Begin by understanding the unique needs of your family members based on their age, sex, health status, and lifestyle. For instance, children's health metrics differ vastly from adults and need to be tracked accordingly.

The following set of standard health metrics can be beneficial: * BMI: A quick measure of weight against height, BMI reveals if a person is underweight, healthy weight, overweight, or obese. It's a useful indicator of potential health risks related to being overweight. * Blood Pressure: High blood pressure, also known as hypertension, is a warning signal for potential heart-related issues. * Heart Rate: Regular monitoring of resting heart rate offers insights into cardiovascular health. * Blood Tests: Routine blood work assessing parameters like blood glucose, cholesterol levels, vitamin levels, etc., provides a comprehensive health view. * Stamina: Often discerned through exercise tests, stamina gauges one's cardiovascular fitness.

Remember, these are baseline parameters. Depending on family members' specific needs, other metrics like bone density, eye health evaluations, or mental health assessments could also be incorporated.

11.3. Getting The Family Involved

Having a family approach to health assessment promises better involvement and commitment. Here are few techniques to effectively involve your family:

- Make Health a Family Conversation: Normalize talking about health and wellness at home. Encourage discussions, queries, and sharing of information.

- Involvement in Health Evaluations: Arrange for family visits to healthcare providers. This promotes understanding and cohesiveness.

- Shared Family Goals: Collective health goals keep the motivation high and can facilitate friendly competition.

- Communicate Achievements: Sharing individual and family achievements encourages continued efforts.

11.4. Charting Progress

Once baseline measurements are set, progress tracking becomes vital. Regular tracking lets you understand the effectiveness of your wellness efforts, identify patterns, and make necessary interventions.

A simple tracking sheet could look like this:

```
|===
| Name | Age | BMI | Blood Pressure | Heart Rate |
Stamina Measurement
| John Doe | 35 | 26 | 120/80 | 70 bpm | 10 mins
| Jane Doe | 33 | 23 | 110/70 | 70 bpm | 12 mins
| Little Doe | 7 | 17 | NA | 85 bpm | NA
|===
```

The frequency of these measurements vary. While BMI could be measured monthly, blood tests might be annual, depending on your healthcare provider's advice.

11.5. From Measurement to Motivation

Monitoring your family's health progress shouldn't be drudgery but a motivation fountain. Here are a few strategies:

- Inculcate a Progress Mindset: Emphasize that 'progress' doesn't mean perfection. Health is a journey, not a destination. Celebrate every small improvement.

- Encourage Without Overburdening: Too much focus on health metrics can potentially induce anxiety. Balancing encouragement with empathy is crucial.

- Use Visual Aids: Use progress charts, graphs, or apps to visualize improvements. These aids boost morale and give a tangible sense of accomplishment.

- Rewards and Incentives: Healthy rewards or incentives can be valuable motivational tools. They can range from a family outing to a new book or gadget.

11.6. Consistency is Key

Consistency fuels progress. Without regular monitoring and effort, maintaining health advancements becomes challenging. Here, routine and discipline play crucial roles.

- Routine Formation: Incorporating health-screenings into your family routine ensures regularity.

- Reinforcing Discipline: Set norms and maintain discipline, especially with kids. This could mean fixed bedtimes, screen times or mandatory physical activities.

- Flexibility: There can be variations and deviations in any routine. Embrace them; they're opportunities to teach about resilience and adaptability.

In conclusion, charting your family's health progress involves measurement, motivation, and consistency. It is a long-term commitment and an evolving process. Understanding the importance of health measurement, setting health metrics, getting the family involved, charting progress, and maintaining consistency form core elements of this process. The wellness journey should embrace progress over perfection while serving as an enjoyable educational experience. After all, the family that stays fit together, lives well together!